Air Fryer Cookbook Recipes for Busy People

Quick and Fast Side Dish Recipes to Make Everyday Meals Taste Better

Samiyah Pearson

© **Copyright 2021 - All rights reserved.**

The content contained within this book may not be reproduced, duplicated or transmitted without direct written permission from the author or the publisher.

Under no circumstances will any blame or legal responsibility be held against the publisher, or author, for any damages, reparation, or monetary loss due to the information contained within this book. Either directly or indirectly.

Legal Notice:

This book is copyright protected. This book is only for personal use. You cannot amend, distribute, sell, use, quote or paraphrase any part, or the content within this book, without the consent of the author or publisher.

Disclaimer Notice:

Please note the information contained within this document is for educational and entertainment purposes only. All effort has been executed to present accurate, up to date, and reliable, complete information. No warranties of any kind are declared or implied. Readers acknowledge that the author is not engaging in the rendering of legal, financial, medical or professional advice. The content within this book has been derived from various sources. Please consult a licensed professional before attempting any techniques outlined in this book.

By reading this document, the reader agrees that under no circumstances is the author responsible for any losses, direct or indirect, which are incurred as a result of the use of information contained within this document, including, but not limited to, — errors, omissions, or inaccuracies.

Table of contents

CILANTRO BRUSSELS SPROUTS 7
GARLIC BEETS 9
GINGER MUSHROOMS 10
MASALA POTATOES 12
LIME BROCCOLI 13
CAJUN ASPARAGUS 14
SQUASH SALAD 16
CREAMY SQUASH MIX 17
ORANGE CARROTS 19
TOMATO SALAD 21
TOMATO AND GREEN BEANS SALAD 23
BELL PEPPERS AND KALE 24
GARLIC PARSNIPS 26
BROCCOLI AND POMEGRANATE 27
BACON CAULIFLOWER 29
PANEER CHEESE BALLS 30
RUSSET POTATO HAY 32
ONION RINGS 34
BREADED AVOCADO FRIES 37
BUFFALO CHICKEN STRIPS 40
SWEET POTATO CHIPS 43
SWEET POTATO TOTS 46
CORN NUTS 49
TEMPURA VEGETABLES 52
SHRIMP A LA BANG SAUCE 56
ZUCCHINIS AND WALNUTS 59
CORIANDER ARTICHOKES 60
TASTY EGGPLANT SLICES 62
BABA GHANOUSH 64
HEALTHY BEET HUMMUS 67
CHICKEN JALAPENO POPPER DIP 70
ROASTED EGGPLANT 72
SPINACH DIP 74
SPICED CAULIFLOWER 77
ROASTED TOMATOES 79
ROASTED RED PEPPER HUMMUS 81
ROASTED FENNEL 84
RADISHES AND SESAME SEEDS 86

HERBED RADISH SAUTÉ.. 88

SAUSAGE MUSHROOM CAPS.. 90

SPANAKOPITA MINIS.. 93

GREEK FETA FRIES OVERLOAD.. 96

SOUR CREAM MUSHROOMS.. 98

RICED CAULIFLOWER BALLS.. 100

ALL-CRISP SWEET POTATO SKINS 103

CREAMY CAULIFLOWER DIP.. 106

CHICKEN BACON BITES 108

6

Cilantro Brussels Sprouts

Serves: 4

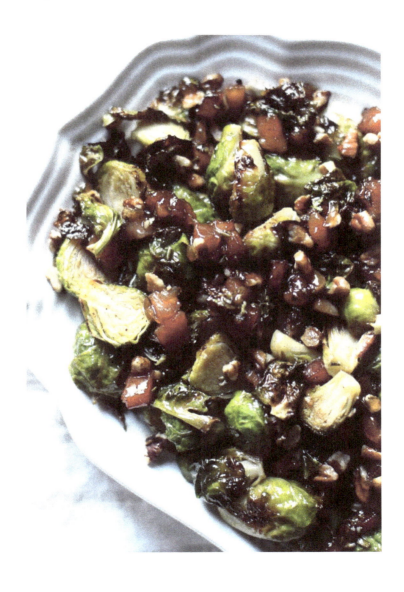

- pounds Brussels sprouts, trimmed and halved 1 tablespoon olive oil

- 2 tablespoons maple syrup

- tablespoon cilantro, chopped 1 tablespoon sweet paprika

- A pinch of salt and black pepper

1.In your air fryer's basket, combine the sprouts with the oil, maple syrup and the remaining , toss and cook at 360 degrees f for 25 minutes.

2.Divide between plates and serve as a side dish.

Garlic Beets

Serves: 4

- pounds beets, peeled and roughly cubed A pinch of salt

  and black pepper

- teaspoon chili powder 4 garlic cloves, minced 1

  tablespoon olive oil

  1.In your air fryer's basket, combine the beets with salt,

  pepper and

  2.the other , toss and cook at 370 degrees f for 25 minutes.

  3.Divide the beets between plates and serve as a side dish.

Ginger Mushrooms

Serves: 4

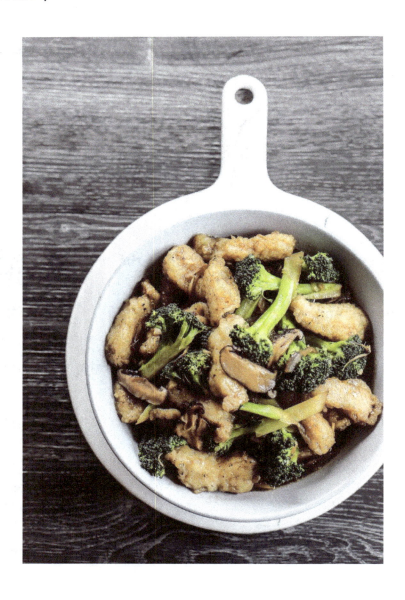

- tablespoons olive oil

- 2 tablespoons balsamic vinegar

- 2 pounds white mushrooms, halved 1 tablespoon ginger, grated

- A pinch of salt and black pepper 1 teaspoon cumin, ground

1.In your air fryer's basket, combine the mushrooms with the oil, vinegar and the other , toss and cook at 360 degrees f for 20 minutes.

2.Divide the mix between plates and serve.

Masala Potatoes

Serves: 4

- pounds gold potatoes, peeled and roughly cubed

  - tablespoon olive oil

  - 1 teaspoon garlic powder 1 teaspoon germ masala

    Juice of 1 lime

  - A pinch of salt and black pepper

1.In your air fryer's basket, combine the potatoes with the

garam masala and the other , toss and cook at 370 degrees

f for 20 minutes.

2.Divide the mix between plates and serve.

Lime Broccoli

Serves: 4

- tablespoon avocado oil

- 1-pound broccoli florets

- 1 tablespoon ginger, grated

- A pinch of salt and black pepper Juice of 1 lime

1.In your air fryer's basket, combine the broccoli with the oil and the other , toss and cook at 370 degrees f for 20 minutes.

2.Divide the mix between plates and serve.

Cajun Asparagus

Serves: 4

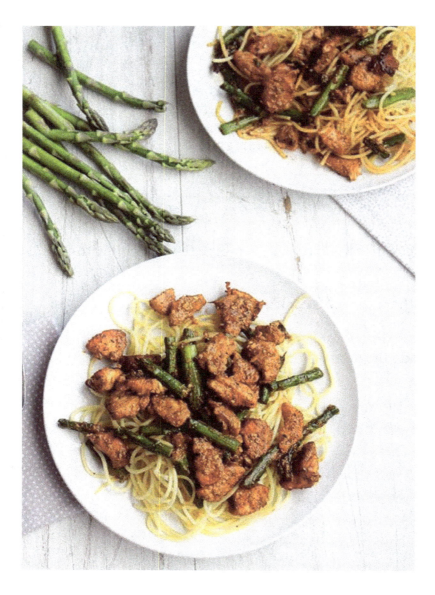

- teaspoon extra virgin olive oil

- 1 bunch asparagus, trimmed

- ½ tablespoon Cajun seasoning

1. In a bowl, mix the asparagus with the oil and Cajun seasoning; coat the asparagus well.

2. Put the asparagus in your air fryer and cook at 400 degrees f for 5

3. minutes.

4. Divide between plates and serve.

Squash Salad

Serves: 4

- butternut squash, cubed

- tablespoons balsamic vinegar 1 bunch cilantro, chopped

- Salt and black pepper to taste 1 tablespoon olive oil

1.Put the squash in your air fryer, and add the salt, pepper, and

oil; toss well.

2.Cook at 400 degrees f for 12 minutes.

3.Transfer the squash to a bowl, add the vinegar and cilantro,

and toss.

4.Serve and enjoy!

Creamy Squash Mix

Serves: 6

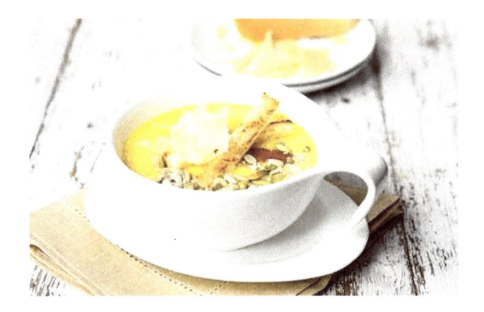

- big butternut squash, roughly cubed

- 1 cup sour cream

- Salt and black pepper to taste

- 1 tablespoon parsley, chopped

- A drizzle of olive oil

1.Put the squash in your air fryer, add the salt and pepper, and

rub with the oil.

2.Cook at 400 degrees f for 12 minutes.

3.Transfer the squash to a bowl, and add the cream and the

parsley.

4.Toss and serve.

Orange Carrots

Serves: 4

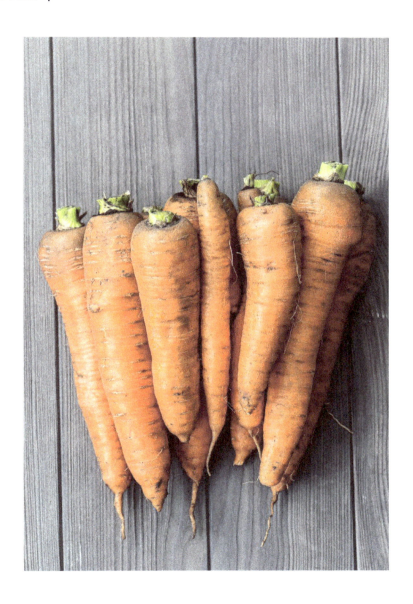

- 1½ pounds baby carrots

- 2 teaspoons orange zest

- tablespoons cider vinegar

- ½ cup orange juice

- A handful of parsley, chopped A drizzle of olive oil

1.Put the baby carrots in your air fryer's basket, add the orange zest and oil, and rub the carrots well.

2.Cook at 350 degrees f for 15 minutes.

3.Transfer the carrots to a bowl, and then add the vinegar, orange juice, and parsley.

4.Toss, serve, and enjoy!

Tomato Salad

Serves: 8

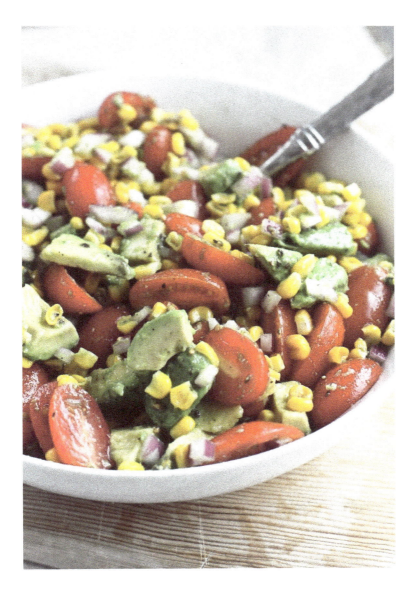

- red onion, sliced

- ounces feta cheese, crumbled

- Salt and black pepper to taste

- 1 pint mixed cherry tomatoes, halved

- 2 ounces pecans

- tablespoons olive oil

-

1.In your air fryer, mix the tomatoes with the salt, pepper, onions, and the oil.

2.Cook at 400 degrees f for 5 minutes.

3. Transfer to a bowl and add the pecans and the cheese.

4.Toss and serve.

Tomato And Green Beans Salad

Serves: 4

- 1-pound green beans, trimmed and halved 2 green onions, chopped

- ounces canned green chilies, chopped

- jalapeno pepper, chopped A drizzle of olive oil

- teaspoons chili powder 1 teaspoon garlic powder

- Salt and black pepper to taste

- cherry tomatoes, halved

1.Place all in a pan that fits your air fryer, and mix / toss.

2.Put the pan in the fryer and cook at 400 degrees f for 6 minutes.

3.Divide the mix between plates and serve hot.

Bell Peppers And Kale

Serves: 4

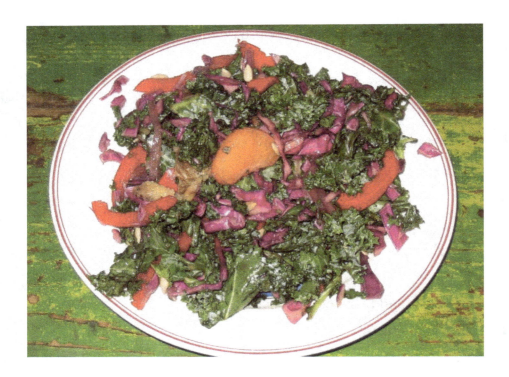

- red bell peppers, cut into strips

- 2 green bell peppers, cut into strips

- ½ pound kale leaves

- Salt and black pepper to taste

- 2 yellow onions, roughly chopped

- ¼ cup veggie stock

- tablespoons tomato sauce

1.Add all to a pan that fits your air fryer; mix well.

2.Place the pan in the fryer and cook at 360 degrees f for 15

minutes.

3.Divide between plates, serve, and enjoy!

Garlic Parsnips

Serves: 4

- 1-pound parsnips, cut into chunks 1 tablespoon olive oil

- garlic cloves, minced

- tablespoon balsamic vinegar Salt and black pepper to

  taste

  1.Add all of the to a bowl and mix well.

  2.Place them in the air fryer and cook at 380 degrees f for

  15 minutes.

  3.Divide between plates and serve.

Broccoli And Pomegranate

Serves: 4

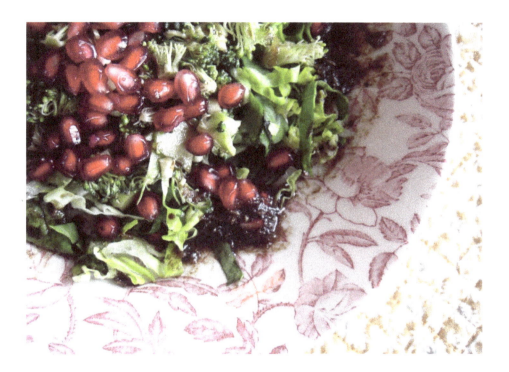

- broccoli head, florets separated

- Salt and black pepper to taste

- 1 pomegranate, seeds separated

- A drizzle of olive oil

1.In a bowl, mix the broccoli with the salt, pepper, and oil; toss.

2.Put the florets in your air fryer and cook at 400 degrees f for 7 minutes.

3.Divide between plates, sprinkle the pomegranate seeds all over, and serve.

Bacon Cauliflower

Serves: 4

- cauliflower head, florets separated 1 tablespoon olive oil

- Salt and black pepper to taste

- ½ cup bacon, cooked and chopped 2 tablespoons dill,

  chopped

1.Put the cauliflower in your air fryer and add the salt, pepper,

and oil; toss well.

2.Cook at 400 degrees f for 12 minutes.

3.Divide the cauliflower between plates, sprinkle the bacon and

the dill on top, and serve.

Paneer Cheese Balls

Serves: 6

- cup paneer, crumbled 1 cup cheese, grated

- 1 potato, boiled and mashed

- 1 onion, chopped finely

- 1 green chili, chopped finely 1 teaspoon red chili flakes

  Salt to taste

- tbsp coriander leaves, chopped finely

- ½ cup all-purpose flour

- ¾ cup of water Breadcrumbs as needed

  1.Mix flour with water in a bowl and spread the

  breadcrumbs in a tray.

  2.Add the rest of the to make the paneer mixture.

3.Make golf ball-sized balls out of this mixture.

4.Dip each ball in the flour liquid then coat with the

breadcrumbs.

5.Place the cheese balls in the instant pot duo and spray it

with Cooking spray.

6.Put on the air fryer lid and seal it.

7.Hit the "air fry button" and select 15 minutes of Cooking

time, then press "start."

8.Once the instant pot duo beeps, remove its lid.

9.Serve.

Russet Potato Hay

Serves: 4

- russet potatoes

- tablespoon olive oil

- Salt and black pepper to taste

1. Pass the potatoes through a spiralizer to get potato spirals.

2.Soak these potato spirals in a bowl filled with water for about

20 minutes.

3.Drain and rinse the soaked potatoes then pat them dry.

4.Toss the potato spirals with salt, black pepper, and oil in a

bowl.

5.Spread the seasoned potato spirals in the air fryer basket.

6.Set this air fryer basket in the instant pot duo.

7.Put on the air fryer lid and seal it.

8.Hit the "air fry button" and select 15 minutes of Cooking time,

then press "start."

9.Toss the potato spiral when halfway cooked then resume

Cooking .

10.once the instant pot duo beeps, remove its lid.

11.serve.

Onion Rings

Serves: 4

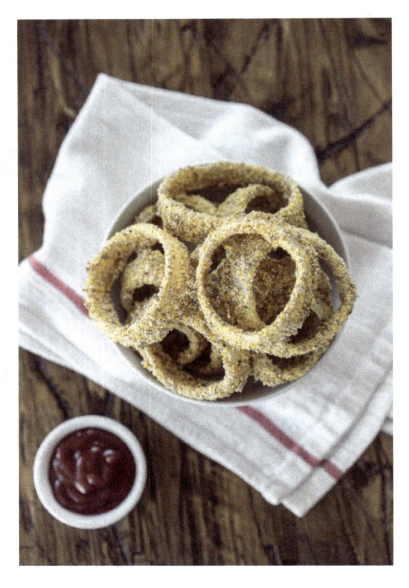

- 3/4 cup flour

- large yellow onion, sliced and rings separated

- ¼ tsp garlic powder

- ¼ tsp paprika

- 1 cup almond milk - 1 large egg 1/2 cup cornstarch

- 1 ½ teaspoons of baking powder 1 teaspoon salt

- 1 cup breadcrumbs

- Cooking spray

1.Whisk flour with baking powder, salt, and cornstarch in a bowl.

2. Coat the onion rings with this dry flour mixture and keep them

aside.

3.Beat egg with milk in a bowl and dip the rings in this mixture.

4.Place the coated rings in the air fryer basket and set it inside

the instant pot duo.

5.Spray the onion rings with Cooking oil. Put on the air fryer lid

and seal it.

6.Hit the "air fry button" and select 10 minutes of Cooking time,

then press "start." Flip the rings when cooked halfway through.

Once the instant pot duo beeps, remove its lid. Serve.

Breaded Avocado Fries

Serves: 4

- 1/4 cup all-purpose flour

- 1/2 teaspoon ground black pepper 1/4 teaspoon salt

- egg

- 1 teaspoon water

- 1 ripe avocado, peeled, pitted and sliced 1/2 cup panko

  breadcrumbs

- Cooking spray

  1.Whisk flour with salt and black pepper in one bowl.

  2.Beat egg with water in another and spread the crumbs in

  a shallow tray.

3.First coat the avocado slices with the flour mixture then dip them into the egg.

4.Drop off the excess and coat the avocado with panko crumbs liberally.

5.Place all the coated slices in the air fryer basket and spray them with Cooking oil.

6.Set the air fryer basket inside the instant pot duo.

7.Put on the air fryer lid and seal it.

8.Hit the "air fry button" and select 7 minutes of Cooking time, then press "start."

9.Flip the fries after 4 minutes of Cooking and resume Cooking .

10. Once the instant pot duo beeps, remove its lid. Serve

fresh.

Buffalo Chicken Strips

Serves:4

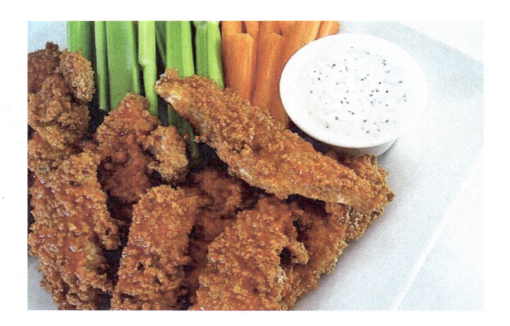

- 1/2 cup Greek yogurt

- 1/4 cup egg

- ½ tablespoon hot sauce

- 1 cup panko breadcrumbs

- 1 tablespoon sweet paprika

- 1 tablespoon garlic pepper seasoning 1 tablespoon cayenne pepper

- 1-pound chicken breasts, cut into strips

1. Mix greek yogurt with hot sauce and egg in a bowl.

2. Whisk breadcrumbs with garlic powder, cayenne pepper, and paprika in another bowl.

3. First, dip the chicken strips in the yogurt sauce then coat them with the crumb's mixture.

4. Place the coated strips in the air fryer basket and spray them with Cooking oil.

5. Set the air fryer basket inside the instant pot duo.

6. Put on the air fryer lid and seal it.

7. Hit the "air fry button" and select 16 minutes of Cooking time, then press "start."

8. Flip the chicken strips after 8 minutes of Cooking then resume air fearing.

9. Once the instant pot duo beeps, remove its lid.

10. Serve.

Sweet Potato Chips

Serves: 2

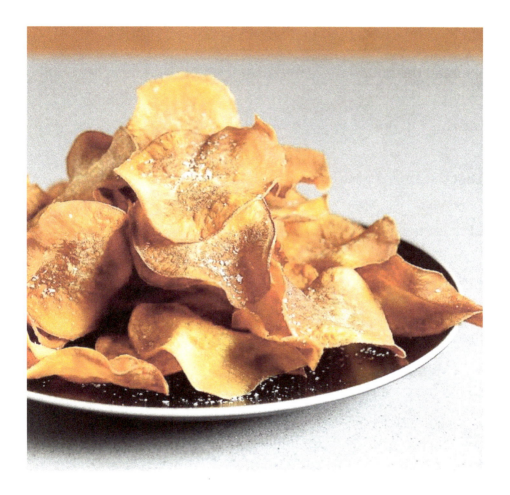

- teaspoon avocado oil

- medium sweet potato, peeled and sliced 1/2 teaspoon

creole seasoning

1.Toss the sweet potato with avocado oil and creole seasoning in

a bowl.

2.Spread the potato slices in the air fryer basket and spray them

with oil.

3.Set the air fryer basket in the instant pot duo.

4.Put on the air fryer lid and seal it.

5.Hit the "air fry button" and select 13 minutes of Cooking time,

then press "start."

6.Toss the potato slices after 7 minutes of Cooking and resume

air

7.frying.

8.Once the instant pot duo beeps, remove its lid.

9.Serve fresh.

Sweet Potato Tots

Serves:4

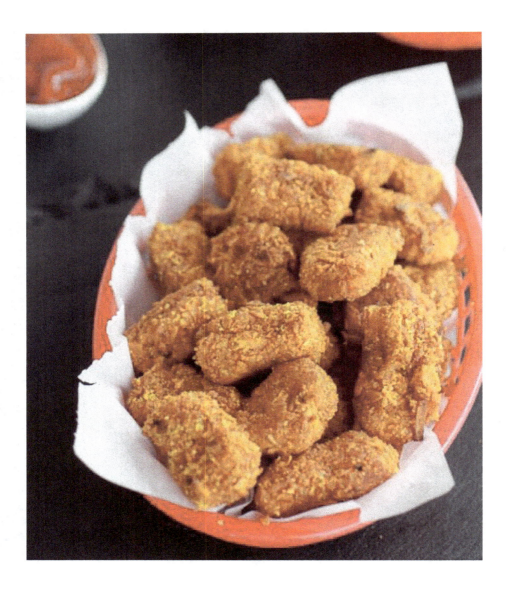

- sweet potatoes, peeled

- 1/2 teaspoon cajun seasoning Olive oil Cooking spray

- Sea salt to taste

1. Add sweet potatoes to boiling water in a pot and cook for 15 minutes until soft.

2. Drain the boiled sweet potatoes and allow them to cool down.

3. Grate the potatoes into a bowl and stir in cajun seasoning and salt.

4. Mix well and make small tater tots out of this mixture.

5. Place these tater tots in the air fryer basket and spray them with Cooking oil.

6. Set the air fryer basket in the instant pot duo.

7.Put on the air fryer lid and seal it.

8.Hit the "air fry button" and select 16 minutes of Cooking

time, then press "start."

9.After 8 minutes, flip all the tots and spray them again

with Cooking oil then resume Cooking .

10.Once the instant pot duo beeps, remove its lid.

11.Serve fresh.

Corn Nuts

Serves:6

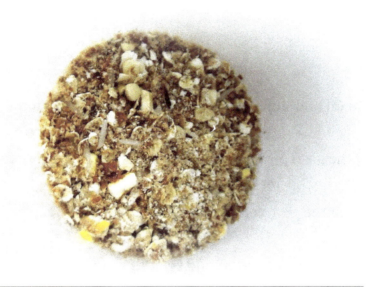

- oz. Giant white corn

- tablespoons vegetable oil 1

- 1/2 teaspoons salt

1.Soak white corn in a bowl filled with water and leave it for 8 hours.

2.Drain the soaked corns and spread them in the air fryer basket.

3.Leave to dry for 20 minutes after patting them dry with a paper towel.

4.Add oil and salt on top of the corns and toss them well.

5.Set the air fryer basket in the instant pot.

6.Put on the air fryer lid and seal it.

7.Hit the "air fry button" and select 20 minutes of Cooking time, then press "start."

8.Shake the corns after every 5 minutes of Cooking , then resume the function.

9.Once the instant pot duo beeps, remove its lid.

10.Serve.

Tempura Vegetables

Serves: 4

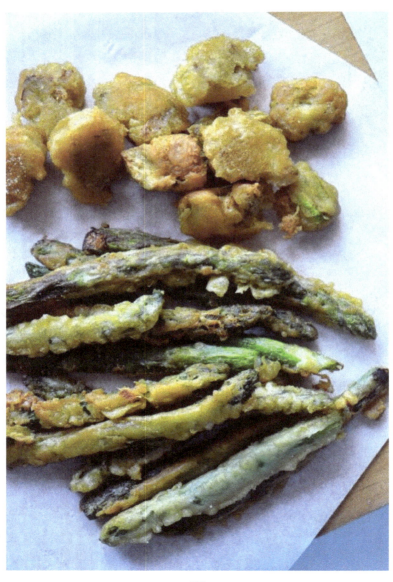

- 1/2 cup all-purpose flour

- 1/2 teaspoon salt, divided, or more to taste

- 1/2 teaspoon ground black pepper

- eggs

- 2 tablespoons water

- cup panko breadcrumbs 2 teaspoons vegetable oil

- 1/2 cup whole green beans

- 1/2 cup asparagus spears

- 1/2 cup red onion rings

- 1/2 cup sweet pepper rings

- 1/2 cup avocado wedges

- 1/2 cup zucchini slices

1. Whisk flour with black pepper and salt in a shallow dish.

2.Beat eggs with water in a bowl and mix panko with oil in another tray.

3.Coat all the veggies with flour mixture first, then dip them in egg and finally in the panko mixture to a coat.

4.Shake off the excess and keep the coated veggies in separate plates.

5.Set half of the coated vegetables in a single layer in the air fryer basket.

6.Place the basket in the instant pot duo and spray them with Cooking oil.

7.Put on the air fryer lid and seal it.

8.Hit the "air fry button" and select 10 minutes of Cooking time, then press "start."

9.Once the instant pot duo beeps, remove its lid.

10.Transfer the fried veggies to the serving plates and

cooking the remaining half using the same steps.

11.Serve.

Shrimp A La Bang Sauce

Serves: 6

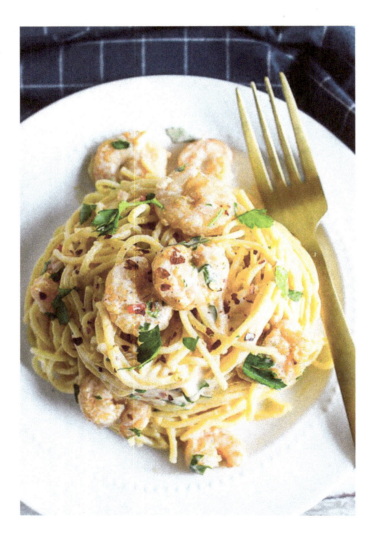

- 1/2 cup mayonnaise

- 1/4 cup sweet chili sauce

- 1 tablespoon Sirach sauce

- 1/4 cup all-purpose flour

- 1 cup panko breadcrumbs

- 1-pound raw shrimp, peeled and deveined

- 1 head loose-leaf lettuce

- green onions, chopped, or to taste

1.Whisk mayonnaise with Sirach, chili sauce in a bowl until smooth.

2.Spread flour in one plate and panko in the other.

3.Place flour on a plate. Place panko on a separate plate.

4.First coat the shrimp with the flour, then dip in

mayonnaise mixture and finally coat with the panko.

5.Arrange the shrimp in the air fryer basket in a single

layer. (do not

6.overcrowd)

7.Set the air fryer basket in the instant pot duo.

8.Put on the air fryer lid and seal it.

9.Hit the "air fry button" and select 12 minutes of Cooking

time, then press "start."

10.Once the instant pot duo beeps, remove its lid.

11.Air fry the remaining shrimp in the same way.

12.Garnish with lettuce and green onion.

13.Serve.

Zucchinis And Walnuts

Serves:4

- lb. Zucchinis; sliced

- ¼ cup chives; chopped.

- cup walnuts; chopped. 4 oz. Arugula leaves

- 1 tbsp. Olive oil

- Salt and white pepper to the taste

1.In a pan that fits the air fryer, combine all the except the

arugula and walnuts, toss, put the pan in the machine and cook

at 360°f for 20 minutes

2.Transfer this to a salad bowl, add the arugula and the walnuts,

toss and serve as a side salad.

Coriander Artichokes

Serves: 4

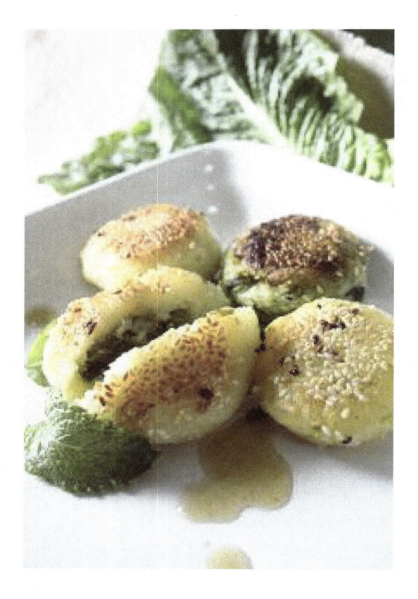

- oz. Artichoke hearts

- 1 tbsp. Lemon juice

- tsp. Coriander, ground

- ½ tsp. Cumin seeds

- ½ tsp. Olive oil

- Salt and black pepper to taste.

1.In a pan that fits your air fryer, mix all the , toss,

introduce the pan in the fryer and cook at 370°f for 15

minutes

2.Divide the mix between plates and serve as a side dish.

Tasty Eggplant Slices

Serves: 4

- eggplant, cut into 1/4-inch thick slices 1/4 tsp garlic powder

- tsp paprika

- 1/4 tsp onion powder

  1.Add all into the mixing bowl and toss until well coated.

  2.Spray the dehydrating tray with Cooking spray and place in instant pot duo crisp air fryer basket.

  3.Arrange eggplant slices on the dehydrating tray.

  4.Place air fryer basket into the pot.

  5.Seal the pot with air fryer lid, select dehydrate mode and cook at 145 f for 4 hours.

6.Serve or store.

Baba Ghanoush

Serves: 6

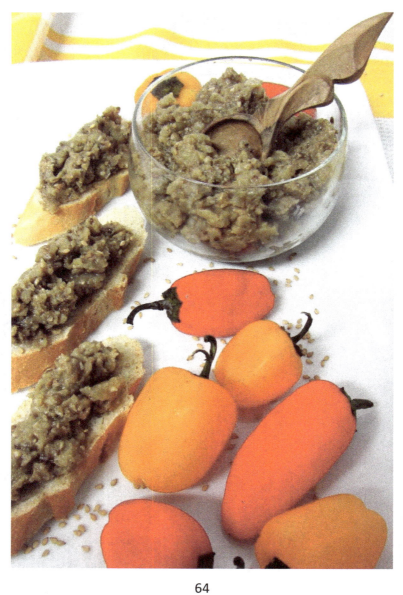

- eggplant, pierce with a fork

- tbsp sesame seeds 2 tbsp sesame oil

- tsp lemon juice

- 1/2 tsp ground cumin

- 1 garlic clove, minced

- 1/2 onion, chopped

- tsp sea salt

  1.Pour 1 cup of water into the inner pot of instant pot duo

  crisp. Place steamer rack in the pot.

  2. Place eggplant on top of the steamer rack.

  3.Seal the pot with pressure Cooking lid and cook on high

  pressure for 8 minutes.

4.Once done, release pressure using a quick release.

Remove lid.

5.Remove eggplant from pot and clean the pot. Peel and

slice cooked eggplant.

6.Add oil into the pot and set a pot on sauté mode.

7.Add onion and eggplant and sauté for 3-5 minutes.

8.Add remaining and stir everything well to combine.

9.Turn off the instant pot. Blend eggplant mixture using

blender until smooth.

10.Serve and enjoy.

Healthy Beet Hummus

Serves: 16

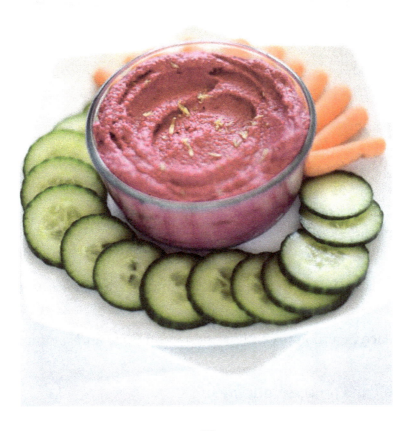

- cup chickpeas 1/3 cup

- water 1/4 cup

- olive oil 1/4 cup

- fresh lemon juice 3 beets,

- peeled and diced 2 garlic cloves,

- peeled 1/4 cup sunflower seeds 1 1/2 tsp kosher salt

  1.Add beets, chickpeas, 1 tsp salt, 3 cups water, garlic, and sunflower seeds into the instant pot.

  2.Seal pot with lid and cook on manual high pressure for 40 minutes.

  3. Strain beet, chickpeas, garlic, and sunflower seeds and place in a food processor and lemon juice and remaining salt and process until smooth.

4.Add oil and 1/3 cup water and process until smooth.

5.Serve and enjoy.

Chicken Jalapeno Popper Dip

Serves: 10

- lb. Chicken breast, boneless 1/2 cup water

- 1/2 cup breadcrumbs 3/4 cup sour cream

- jalapeno pepper, sliced 8 oz cream cheese

- oz cheddar cheese

1.Add chicken, jalapeno, water, and cream cheese into the

instant pot.

2.Seal pot with lid and cook on manual high pressure for 12

minutes.

3.Once done then release pressure using the quick-release

method than open the lid.

4.Stir in cream and cheddar cheese.

5.Transfer instant pot mixture to the baking dish and top with

breadcrumbs and broil for 2 minutes.

6.Serve and enjoy.

Roasted Eggplant

Serves:4

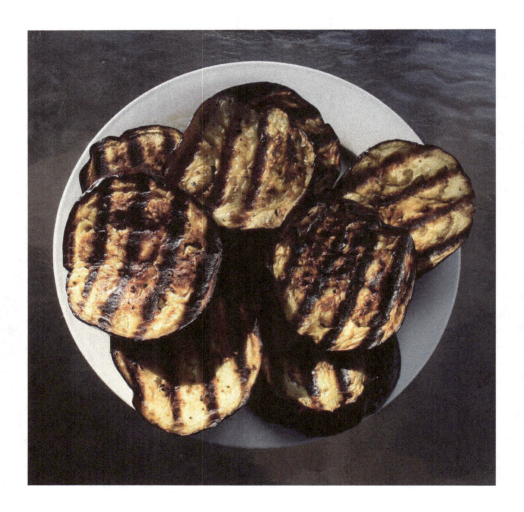

- large eggplant 2 tbsp.

- Olive oil

- ½ tsp. Garlic powder.

- ¼ tsp. Salt

1.Remove top and bottom from eggplant. Slice eggplant into ¼-inchthick round slices.

2.Brush slices with olive oil.

3.Sprinkle with salt and garlic powder

4.Place eggplant slices into the air fryer basket.

5.Adjust the temperature to 390 degrees f and set the timer for 15 minutes.

6.Serve immediately.

Spinach Dip

Serves: 8

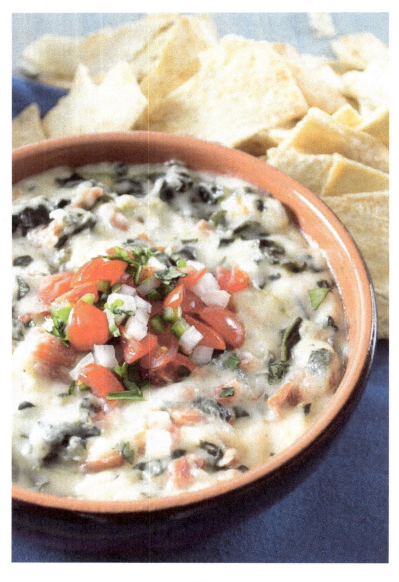

- (8-oz. Package cream cheese, softened

- cup mayonnaise

- 1 cup parmesan cheese, grated

- 1 cup frozen spinach, thawed and squeezed

- 1/3 cup water chestnuts, drained and chopped

- ½ cup onion, minced

- ¼ teaspoon garlic powder Ground black pepper, as required

1. In a bowl, add all the and mix until well combined.

2. Transfer the mixture into a baking pan and spread in an even layer.

3. Press "power button" of air fry oven and turn the dial to select the

4."air fry" mode.

5.Press the time button and again turn the dial to set the

Cooking time to 35 minutes.

6.Now push the temp button and rotate the dial to set the

temperature at 300 degrees f.

7.Press "start/pause" button to start.

8.When the unit beeps to show that it is preheated, open

the lid.

9.Arrange pan over the "wire rack" and insert in the oven.

10.Stir the dip once halfway through.

11.Serve hot.

Spiced Cauliflower

Serves: 4

- cauliflower head, florets separated

- tbsp. Olive oil

- 1 tbsp. Butter; melted

- ¼ tsp. Cinnamon powder

- ¼ tsp. Cloves, ground

- ¼ tsp. Turmeric powder

- ½ tsp. Cumin, ground

- A pinch of salt and black pepper

1.Take a bowl and mix cauliflower florets with the rest of the and

toss.

2. Put the cauliflower in your air fryer's basket and cook at 390°f

for 15 minutes

3.Divide between plates and serve as a side dish.

Roasted Tomatoes

Serves: 4

- tomatoes; halved

- ½ cup parmesan; grated 1 tbsp. Basil; chopped.

- ½ tsp. Onion powder

- ½ tsp. Oregano; dried

- ½ tsp. Smoked paprika

- ½ tsp. Garlic powder Cooking spray

  1.Take a bowl and mix all the except the Cooking spray and the parmesan.

  2.Arrange the tomatoes in your air fryer's pan, sprinkle the parmesan on top and grease with Cooking spray

3.Cook at 370°f for 15 minutes, divide between plates and

serve.

Roasted Red Pepper Hummus

Serves: 4

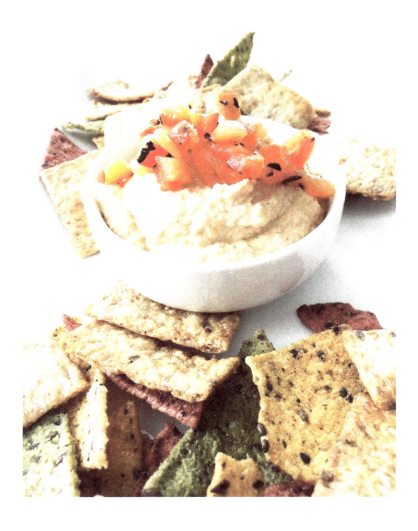

- cup chickpeas, dry and rinsed

- 2 tbsp olive oil

- 1/4 tsp cumin 2 garlic cloves

- 1/2 tbsp tahini

- tbsp fresh lemon juice 1/2 cup roasted red peppers 3 cups chicken broth

- 1/2 tsp salt

1.Add chickpeas and broth into the inner pot of instant pot duo crisp and stir well.

2.Seal the pot with pressure Cooking lid and cook on high for 40 minutes.

3.Once done, allow to release pressure naturally. Remove lid.

4.Drain chickpeas well and reserved half cup broth.

5.Transfer chickpeas, reserved broth, and remaining into the

food processor and process until smooth.

6.Serve and enjoy.

Roasted Fennel

Serves: 4

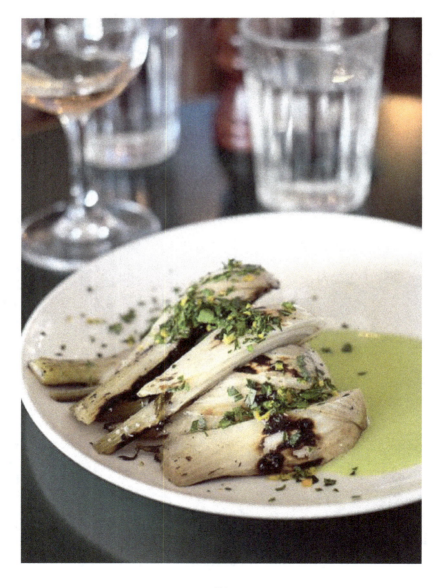

- lb. Fennel; cut into small wedges

- tbsp. Olive oil

- tbsp. Sunflower seeds Juice of ½ lemon

- Salt and black pepper to taste.

1.Take a bowl and mix the fennel wedges with all the

except the sunflower seeds, put them in your air fryer's

basket and cook at 400°f for 15 minutes

2.Divide the fennel between plates, sprinkle the sunflower

seeds on top and serve as a side dish.

Radishes And Sesame Seeds

Serves: 4

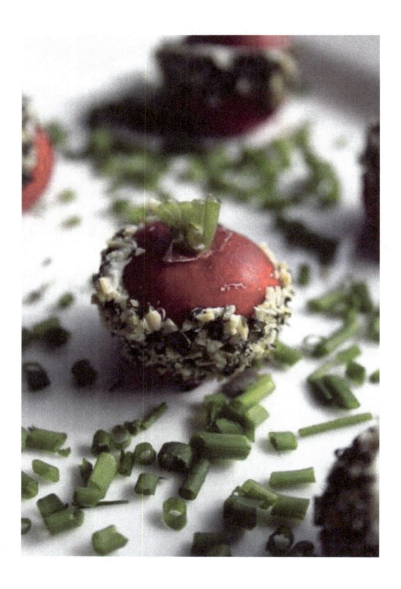

- 20 radishes; halved

- spring onions; chopped.

- 3 green onions; chopped.

- 2 tbsp. Olive oil

- tbsp. Olive oil

- tsp. Black sesame seeds Salt and black pepper to taste.

  1. Take a bowl and mix all the and toss well.

  2. Put the radishes in your air fryer's basket, cook at 400°f for 15 minutes, divide between plates and serve as a side dish

Herbed Radish Sauté

Serves: 4

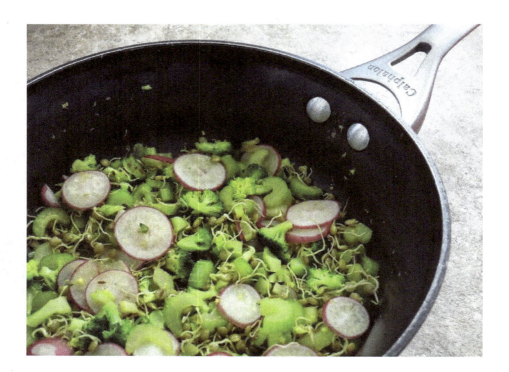

- 2 bunches red radishes; halved

- 2 tbsp. Parsley; chopped.

- 2 tbsp. Balsamic vinegar

- tbsp. Olive oil

- Salt and black pepper to taste.

1.Take a bowl and mix the radishes with the remaining except the parsley, toss and put them in your air fryer's basket.

2. Cook at 400°f for 15 minutes, divide between plates, sprinkle the parsley on top and serve as a side dish

Sausage Mushroom Caps

Serves: 2

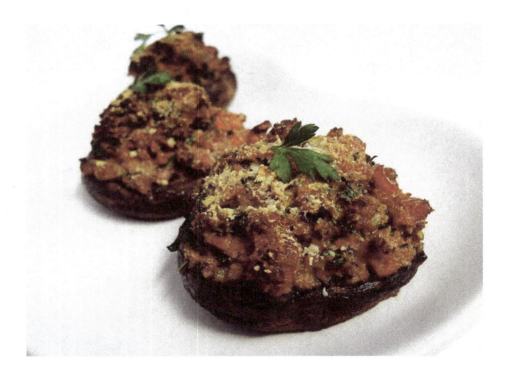

- ½ lb. Italian sausage

- 6 large Portobello mushroom caps

- ¼ cup grated parmesan cheese

- ¼ cup chopped onion

- 2 tbsp. Blanched finely ground almond flour

- 1 tsp. Minced fresh garlic

1. Use a spoon to hollow out each mushroom cap, reserving scrapings.

2. In a medium skillet over medium heat, brown the sausage about 10 minutes or until fully cooked and no pink remains. Drain and then add reserved mushroom scrapings, onion, almond flour, parmesan and garlic.

3. Gently fold together and continue Cooking an additional minute, then remove from heat

4. Evenly spoon the mixture into mushroom caps and place the caps into a 6-inch round pan. Place pan into the air fryer basket

5.Adjust the temperature to 375 degrees f and set the timer

for 8 minutes. When finished Cooking , the tops will be

browned and bubbling. Serve warm.

Spanakopita Minis

Serves: 8

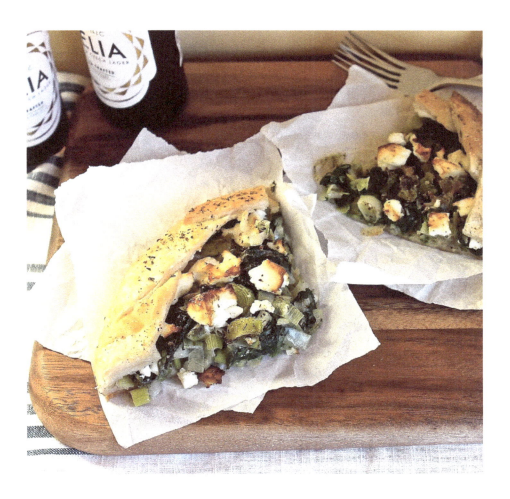

- Olive oil, extra virgin (1 tablespoon)

- Water (2 tablespoons) Egg white, large (1 piece)

- Salt, kosher (1/4 teaspoon)

- Feta cheese, crumbled (1 ounce)

- Oregano, dried (1 teaspoon)

- Phyllo dough, frozen, thawed (4 sheets)

- Baby spinach leaves (10 ounces)

- Cottage cheese, 1% low Fat (1/4 cup)

- Parmesan cheese, grated finely (2 tablespoons)

- Lemon zest, freshly grated (1 teaspoon)

- Black pepper, freshly ground (1/4 teaspoon)

- Cayenne pepper (1/8 teaspoon)

- Cooking spray

1.Boil the spinach in a pot of water; once wilted, drain, cool, and patdry.

2.Add to a bowl filled with egg white, feta cheese, cottage cheese, parmesan cheese, black pepper, cayenne pepper, oregano, lemon zest, and salt; mix well.

3.Brush the phyllo sheets with a little oil before stacking. Cut into 16 equal-sized strips.

4.Add filling (1 tablespoon) onto one of each strip's end before folding the entire phyllo sheet into a triangular packet.

5.Mist Cooking spray onto the air fryer basket. Top with the packets, then mist again with Cooking spray.

6.Cook for twelve minutes at 375 degrees Fahrenheit.

Greek Feta Fries Overload

Serves: 2

- Potatoes, russet/yukon gold, 7-ounce, scrubbed, dried (2 pieces)

- Salt, kosher (1/4 teaspoon)

- Black pepper, freshly ground (1/4 teaspoon) Plum tomatoes, seeded, diced (1/4 cup) Lemon zest, freshly grated (2 teaspoons) Onion powder (1/4 teaspoon)

- Chicken breast, rotisserie, skinless, shredded (2 ounces) Parsley, flat leaf, fresh, chopped (1/2 tablespoon) Oregano, fresh, chopped (1/2 tablespoon)

- Cooking spray

- Olive oil, extra virgin (1 tablespoon) Oregano, dried (1/2 teaspoon) Garlic powder (1/4 teaspoon) Paprika (1/4

teaspoon)

- Feta cheese, grated finely (2 ounces) Tzatziki, prepared

  (1/4 cup)

- Red onion, chopped (2 tablespoons)

1.Set the air fryer at 380 degrees Fahrenheit to preheat.

2.Slice the potatoes into quarter inch-thick fries. Add to a bowl

filled with salt, pepper, onion powder, dried oregano, garlic

powder, paprika, and zest, then toss until well-coated.

3.Cook potato fries in the air fryer for fifteen minutes. Serve

topped with feta cheese, shredded chicken, tzatziki, diced plum

tomatoes, chopped red onion, and fresh herbs.

SOUR CREAM MUSHROOMS

Serves: 24

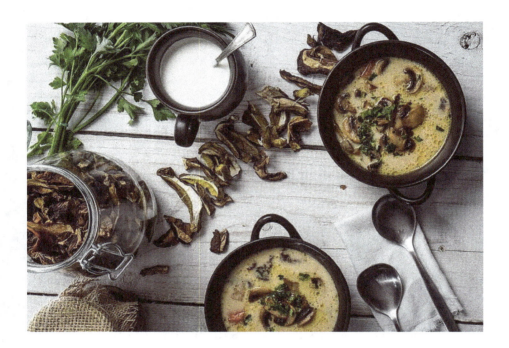

- Bell pepper, orange, diced (1/2 piece) Cheddar cheese, shredded (1 cup) Carrot, small, diced (1 piece)

- Cheddar cheese, shredded (1 ½ tablespoons)

- Mushrooms, w/ stems & caps diced (24 pieces) Onion,

diced (1/2 piece)

- Bacon slices, diced (2 pieces) Sour cream (1/2 cup)

1.Sauté the onion, bacon, mushroom stems, carrot, and orange bell pepper. Once fully cooked, stir in sour cream and cheddar cheese (1 cup) and cook for two minutes Utes.

2.Set the air fryer at 350 degrees Fahrenheit to preheat.

3.Fill mushroom caps with prepared stuffing before topping with remaining cheddar cheese.

4.Cook in the air fryer for eight minutes utes or until cheese melts.

Riced Cauliflower Balls

Serves: 2

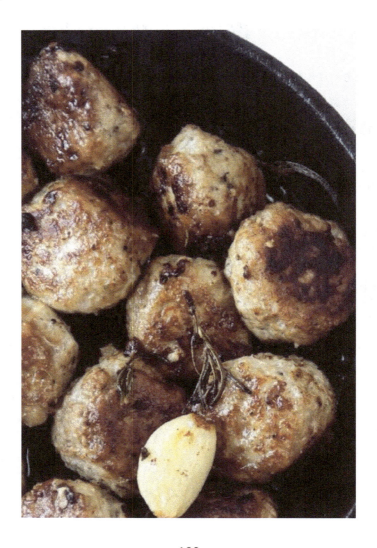

- Cauliflower rice, frozen (2 ¼ cup)

- Egg, large, beaten (1 piece)

- Marinara, homemade (2 tablespoons)

- Cheese, parmesan/pecorino romano, grated (1 tablespoon)

- Chicken sausage, italian, w/ casing removed (1 link) Salt, kosher (1/4 teaspoon)

- Cheese, mozzarella, part skim, shredded (1/2 cup) Breadcrumbs (1/4 cup)

- Cooking spray

1.Cook the sausage on medium-high until cooked through and broken up. Stir in the marinara, salt, and cauliflower and cook for another six minutes utes over medium heat. Turn off heat

before stirring in the mozzarella.

2.Spray the cooled cauliflower mixture with Cooking spray

before molding into 6 balls. Dip each ball in the beaten egg

before coating with breadcrumbs. Load in the air fryer, coat with

Cooking spray, and cook for four to five minutes utes on each

side at 400 degrees fahrenheit.

All-Crisp Sweet Potato Skins

Serves: 6

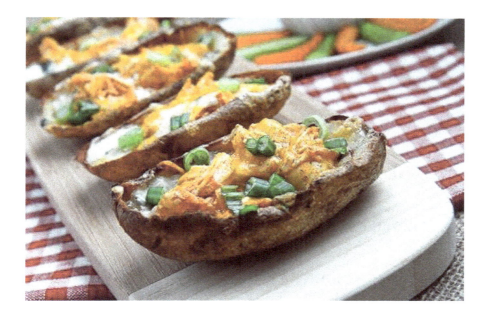

- SCal lions, sliced thinly (2 pieces)

- Cooking spray, olive oil

- Black beans, Fat free, re-fried (1 cup)

- Salt, kosher (1/4 teaspoon)

- Cheese, cheddar, reduced Fat, shredded (3/4 cup)

- Sweet potatoes, small (6 pieces)

- Taco seasoning (1/2 tablespoon)

- Black pepper, freshly ground (1/4 teaspoon) Salsa (3/4 cup)

- Cilantro, chopped (1 tablespoon)

  1. Set the air fryer at 370 degrees fahrenheit to preheat.

  2. Cover the sweet potatoes in parchment and cook in the air fryer for thirty minutes utes. Let cool.

  3. Mix the taco seasoning and black beans.

  4. Halve the cooled sweet potatoes and remove most of the flesh. Spray the skins with Cooking spray, sprinkle with pepper and salt, and air-fry for two to three minutes utes.

5.Fill each skin with black beans, salsa (1 tablespoon), and

cheese (1 tablespoon). Return to the air fryer and cook for

two minutes utes.

6.Serve topped with cilantro and sCal lions.

CREAMY CAULIFLOWER DIP

Serves: 10

- Green onions, chopped (4 pieces)

- Olive oil, extra virgin (2 tablespoons)

- Worcestershire sauce (1 teaspoon)

- Mayonnaise (3/4 cup)

- Parmesan cheese, shredded (1 ½ cups)

- Cauliflower head (1 piece)

- Cream cheese, softened (8 ounces)

- Sour cream (1/2 cup)

- Garlic cloves (2 pieces)

1. Break the cauliflower into florets after washing and

patting dry. Toss with olive oil until evenly coated.

2.Place florets in the air fryer and cook for twenty minutes utes at 390 degrees fahrenheit, turning halfway.

3.Transfer the roasted florets into the blender and process with the sour cream, cream cheese, parmesan cheese (1 cup), mayonnaise, green onions, garlic, and worcestershire sauce.

4.Pour the blended cauliflower mixture into a bake dish (7x7-inch) and top with the remaining parmesan cheese. Cook in the air fryer for ten to fifteen minutes utes at 360 degrees fahrenheit.

Chicken Bacon Bites

Serves: 4

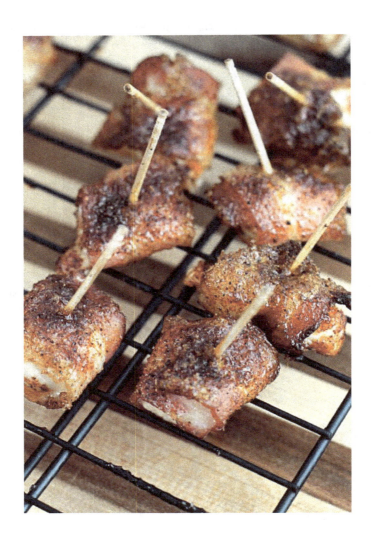

- Bacon slices, cut into 1/3-portions (6 pieces) C

- hili powder (1/2 tablespoon)

- Chicken breast, sliced into one-inch chunks (1 pound)

- Brown Sugar (1/3 cup)

- Cayenne pepper (1/8 teaspoon)

1.Stick a bacon piece onto a chicken piece, then roll to secure,

2.finishing by piercing with a toothpick. Repeat with the

remaining bacon and chicken pieces.

3.Mix the brown Sugar, cayenne pepper, and chili powder and

season the chicken bacon bites.

4.Cook in the air fryer for fifteen minutes utes at 390 degrees f